HERBAL REMEDIES FOR BLOOD SUGAR

Unlocking Nature's Healing Power; Dive Into Effective Remedies, Focus On Holistic Wellness, And Key Strategies For A Healthier Life

DR. CARDEN KYRIE

DISCLAIMER

The only goal of this book is informational. Every effort has been taken by the author and publisher to ensure that the information provided is accurate. But the material in this book is given "as is," without any express or implied representation, warranty, or condition as to its accuracy, completeness, or suitability for any particular purpose.

Any loss, damage, or injury resulting from using the information in this book, or from any action or decision made as a result of such use, will not be covered by the author's or publisher's liability. It is recommended that readers seek the assistance of a certified specialist for guidance specific to their situation.

The opinions and viewpoints conveyed in this book belong to the author and may not necessarily represent the official stance or policies of any specified organizations or people. Any likeness to real-life occurrences, places, or people—living or deceased—is wholly coincidental.

No specific product, service, or therapy discussed in this book is endorsed by the author or publisher. Any reference to goods or services is made only for informative reasons and is not intended as a recommendation or endorsement.

Before making any judgments or acting on any information, readers are urged to independently confirm it all. Any unfavorable effects or repercussions arising from the usage of the material included in this book are disclaimed by the author and publisher.

By using this book, you consent to absolving the publisher and author of any and all claims, obligations, or losses resulting from your use of the material in it.

I appreciate your cooperation and understanding.

TABLE OF CONTENTS

CHAPTER ONE

INTRODUCTION TO BLOOD SUGAR

THE SIGNIFICANCE OF BLOOD SUGAR CONTROL

Sustaining ideal blood sugar levels is essential for general health and wellness, as it forms the basis for the body's correct operation. It is impossible to overestimate the significance of blood sugar regulation because it is essential to many physiological functions, such as hormone balance, organ function, and energy metabolism. To maintain a delicate balance and avoid hyperglycemia (high blood sugar) and hypoglycemia (low blood sugar), the body strictly controls blood sugar levels. Ineffective blood sugar control increases the risk of developing major health issues like diabetes, heart disease, and metabolic disorders. It is therefore crucial to comprehend and give priority to the mechanisms that control blood sugar levels to encourage a robust and healthy lifestyle.

SYNOPSIS OF HERBAL TREATMENTS

For millennia, herbal treatments have been an essential part of traditional medical procedures in various cultures. The idea that nature offers a wide range of compounds with therapeutic qualities is the foundation of the use of herbs for medical purposes. Growing awareness of the potential benefits of herbal treatments and the need for natural alternatives to conventional drugs have led to a resurgence of interest in them in recent times. A wide variety of plants and substances derived from plants are used in herbal medicines; each has special qualities that enhance the therapeutic effects of the remedy. These treatments frequently provide a holistic approach to healthcare, boosting general well-being in addition to treating particular problems. Investigating the field of herbal medicines might lead to prospective opportunities for complementary and integrative healthcare methods as well as insightful understandings of traditional knowledge systems.

In the realm of alternative medicine, there is growing interest in the relationship between blood sugar management and herbal medicines. Some herbs have shown promise in regulating blood sugar levels through the enhancement of insulin sensitivity, the promotion of glucose absorption, or the modulation of insulin secretion from the pancreas. Investigating these herbs' possible function in treating diseases like diabetes or metabolic syndrome begins with an understanding of the mechanisms by which they interact with the body's glucose metabolism. Furthermore, compared to pharmaceutical interventions, herbal therapies frequently have fewer side effects, which makes them a desirable choice for people looking for safer, more natural ways to support their health.

We examine the complex interactions between the significance of blood sugar management and the summary of herbal treatments in this investigation. We hope to shed light on any potential synergies that may exist in using nature's power to support optimal health by looking at the importance of keeping blood sugar levels balanced and the wide range of herbal therapies. This voyage emphasizes a holistic view of well-being that incorporates both conventional and alternative methods for an all-encompassing and well-rounded healthcare plan. It also asks us to recognize the wisdom ingrained in traditional healing practices.

CHAPTER TWO
COMPREHENDING BLOOD SUGAR
SUGAR

Controlling blood sugar levels is essential for preserving general health and well-being. Fundamentally, blood sugar, also known as blood glucose, is the amount of glucose that is in the blood. Since glucose is the body's main energy source for cells, it must be properly regulated for physiological processes to occur. Insulin is a key player in the intricate system of hormones that regulate blood sugar levels, which is a delicate equilibrium.

INSULIN

The production of insulin by the pancreas is an essential component in blood sugar regulation. In response to elevated blood glucose levels, such as following a meal, insulin is produced to promote glucose uptake by cells. This procedure guarantees that cells obtain the energy required for their diverse operations. However, as blood sugar levels fall, the liver is prompted to convert stored glycogen into glucose by the pancreas' production of glucagon, which keeps blood sugar levels within a normal range.

NORMAL LEVELS OF BLOOD SUGAR

Sufficient blood sugar levels are essential for the organs and tissues of the body to operate correctly. Blood sugar levels during fasting usually fall between 70 to 100 mg/dL, while levels after meals, or postprandial, may rise briefly before returning to the fasting range in a few hours. It is crucial to keep these levels within the usual range to avoid long-term health issues as well as temporary pain.

RESULTING FROM AN UNBALANCED BLOOD SUGAR

When blood sugar levels fall outside of the usual range, some consequences might result in hyperglycemia and hypoglycemia. Elevated blood sugar levels, or hyperglycemia, are frequently linked to diabetes mellitus. Long-term high blood sugar levels can harm organs and blood vessels, which can result in consequences like kidney damage, nerve damage, and cardiovascular disease.

LOW BLOOD SUGAR

On the other hand, hypoglycemia happens when blood sugar falls below the normal range, usually less than 70 mg/dL. This illness may be brought on by things like taking too much insulin, missing meals, or exercising vigorously without enough nutrition. Symptoms of hypoglycemia include shakiness, disorientation, and, in extreme cases, unconsciousness. It is imperative to take prompt action to return blood sugar levels to normal, usually by consuming meals or beverages high in glucose.

Realizing the critical roles that glucose and insulin play in preserving physiological balance is essential to comprehend the fundamentals of blood sugar. The body needs normal blood sugar levels to function properly, and abnormalities can have serious repercussions. The extremes of hyperglycemia and hypoglycemia emphasize how crucial it is to keep blood sugar levels within a specific, ideal range for general health and well-being.

CHAPTER THREE

THE EFFECTS OF HERBS ON BLOOD SUGAR

HERBS' PLACE IN CONVENTIONAL MEDICINE

Herbal medicine has been used for a very long time in many different cultures all over the world. Herbal medicine has been utilized by traditional healers to treat a range of health issues, including blood sugar regulation. The long history of using herbs in traditional medicine is indicative of a profound knowledge of the natural world and how it might benefit human health.

BASIS OF HERBAL REMEDIES IN SCIENCE

Scientific studies have recently focused on the complex processes via which herbs affect the human body. The plethora of bioactive chemicals found in these plants provides the scientific foundation for herbal therapies.

These substances, which include alkaloids, polyphenols, and flavonoids, have been found to have insulin-sensitizing, anti-inflammatory, and antioxidant qualities. Gaining knowledge about the biochemical processes by which these substances interact with the body will help you better understand the possible advantages of herbs for blood sugar regulation.

It is important to select herbs for blood sugar management based on scientific studies that have shown their effectiveness. There has been research on the possibility of herbs including ginseng, fenugreek, cinnamon, and bitter melon lowering blood sugar levels. For example, bitter melon has substances that function similarly to insulin, enhancing the uptake of glucose by cells.

Cinnamon has been demonstrated to increase insulin sensitivity, while fenugreek may help control blood sugar by slowing down the absorption of carbohydrates.

SELECTING THE PROPER HERBS TO MANAGE BLOOD SUGAR

Individual tastes, potential adverse effects, and combinations with other treatments should all be considered while selecting herbs. Getting advice from a trained herbalist or medical practitioner can assist in customizing a herbal regimen to fit a person's unique needs and health situation.

It is critical to understand that, despite their potential benefits, herbal remedies for diabetes and other blood sugar-related disorders should never take the place of traditional medical care. Instead, they can support an all-encompassing holistic approach to health by enhancing currently available therapies.

Research into the potential of herbs for blood sugar regulation has been made possible by their use in traditional medicine. Herbs include bioactive chemicals that present a promising option for blood sugar management; research is still ongoing to determine the precise mechanisms of action.

To optimize the advantages of herbs and provide a comprehensive approach to health and well-being, careful selection based on individual factors and scientific evidence is essential when adding them to a blood sugar control program.

CHAPTER FOUR

SAFETY AND PRECAUTIONS

MEDICATIONS AND POSSIBLE INTERACTIONS

To protect people's health, safety concerns about possible drug interactions are essential. Combining some drugs can have negative effects that reduce their therapeutic benefits or possibly cause harm. People must tell medical professionals about everything they take, including prescription, over-the-counter, and dietary supplements. Healthcare practitioners can evaluate the possibility of interactions and decide on treatment regimens with this information at their disposal.

Recognizing such interactions requires an understanding of the pharmacological characteristics of drugs. When two or more medications interfere with one another's body's absorption, metabolism, distribution, or excretion, drug-drug interactions can happen. This may lead to changed therapeutic outcomes or a higher chance of adverse reactions. To promote proactive monitoring of potential interactions, patients should be made aware of the significance of promptly notifying their healthcare providers of any changes in their prescription regimen.

ALLERGIC REACTIONS

The degree and presentation of allergic reactions to drugs and other substances can differ greatly. People must be on the lookout for possible allergic reactions and notify their healthcare professionals right away if they have any strange symptoms. Anaphylaxis, breathing difficulties, skin rashes, swelling, and itching are typical symptoms of an allergic reaction. Allergy reactions can be fatal in extreme circumstances.

If advised by their healthcare physician, people should have allergy testing done before starting any new drug or treatment. This facilitates the identification of possible allergies and the creation of a secure and efficient treatment strategy. When faced with an emergency, like an anaphylactic reaction, people should get medical help right away and, if directed, carry an epinephrine auto-injector.

BIRTH CONTROL WITH HERBAL MEDICINES

When considering herbal medicines, pregnant women should proceed with caution as some compounds may be harmful to the developing fetus. There has been little research on the effects of herbal treatments, therefore their safety during pregnancy is sometimes unknown. To protect the health of the mother and the unborn child, pregnant women should always speak with their healthcare practitioners before using any herbal supplements or therapies.

Certain herbs may interact with hormone processes or have uterine-stimulating properties, which could cause problems during pregnancy. To balance the possible advantages and risks, it is crucial to have open lines of communication with medical specialists. In some cases, safer alternatives may be suggested.

CONSULTATION WITH MEDICAL SPECIALISTS

To guarantee the safety and effectiveness of any medical intervention, consulting with healthcare specialists is essential. Patients and their healthcare providers should have open and honest communication about the patient's medical history, symptoms, and any worries they may have. Healthcare providers can make well-informed judgments that are customized to each patient's unique needs because of this collaborative approach.

People should speak with experts or their primary care providers before beginning any new treatment. Given that the safety and effectiveness of complementary or alternative medicines may not be fully established, this is particularly crucial.

CHAPTER FIVE

TYPICAL HERBS FOR MANAGING BLOOD SUGAR

CINNAMON

The inner bark of plants of the Cinnamomum genus is the source of cinnamon, which has drawn interest due to its potential to control blood sugar. Improving insulin sensitivity and lowering insulin resistance are part of the mechanism of action. A crucial ingredient, cinnamaldehyde, activates insulin receptors and promotes cells' absorption of glucose. Cinnamon may also inhibit specific enzymes that postpone the digestion of carbs, which aids in blood sugar regulation. Although each person reacts differently, a daily dose of 1 to 6 grams, divided into smaller amounts, is generally advised for people looking to benefit their blood sugar levels.

FENUGREEK

The adaptable herb fenugreek has both culinary and therapeutic uses. It has been linked to several health advantages, including the control of blood sugar. It has soluble fiber, which reduces the rate at which sugars and carbohydrates are absorbed, improving blood sugar regulation. Furthermore, the anti-diabetic qualities of fenugreek seeds may be attributed to their abundance of substances like trigonelline. For fenugreek supplements, the suggested daily dosage is usually between 2.5 and 15 grams, split into two or three doses. Fenugreek is well-known for its ability to assist lactation, lower inflammation, and improve digestion in addition to its involvement in blood sugar regulation.

BITTER MELON

Due to its characteristics, bitter melon is being studied as a potential blood sugar management tool. It is frequently used in traditional medicine. It contains polypeptide-p, plant insulin that may help lower blood sugar levels, and charantin, which has actions similar to those of insulin. Additionally high in antioxidants and with anti-inflammatory qualities is bitter melon. The bitter flavor of bitter melon is an acquired preference, and its culinary applications are diverse among cultures. You can include bitter melon in your diet by juicing, stir-frying, or souping it up. Beyond controlling blood sugar, it may also strengthen the immune system and enhance skin health.

SYLVESTRE GYMNEMA

The plant Gymnema sylvestre, which is indigenous to Africa and India, has long been used to treat diabetes. It functions by preventing the intestines from absorbing sugar and encouraging the pancreatic tissue that produces insulin to regenerate. The herb's active ingredients, known as gymnemic acids, are thought to be the cause of its anti-diabetic properties. Gymnema Sylvestre may lower blood sugar levels and reduce the absorption of sugar, according to research findings. Although the suggested dosage varies, popular ranges are 200–800 mg/day split into two or three doses. Before including Gymnema Sylvestre in a diabetic care plan, it is imperative to speak with a healthcare provider, particularly for people who are currently taking medication to control their blood sugar.

Each of these common herbs Bitter Melon, Fenugreek, Cinnamon, and Gymnema Sylvestre offers special mechanisms and qualities in the management of blood sugar. Although encouraging, people with diabetes or those at risk must speak with medical specialists before making big dietary or supplement changes. Although the effects of using these herbs with a healthy lifestyle and balanced diet may differ from person to person, they may help improve blood sugar regulation. Sophisticated strategies and consistent monitoring are essential for effective blood sugar control.

CHAPTER SIX

RECIPES FOR HERBAL TEAS TO CONTROL BLOOD SUGAR

THE IMPACT OF GREEN TEA ON BLOOD SUGAR

Blood sugar control has shown interest in green tea, which is made from Camellia sinensis leaves. The drink contains a lot of polyphenols, especially catechins, which have been linked to certain health advantages. Epigallocatechin gallate (EGCG), one of the main catechins in green tea, has been investigated for its effects on blood sugar levels.

CATECHINS AND SENSITIVITY TO INSULIN

Improvements in insulin sensitivity have been linked to the catechins found in green tea. Increased sensitivity to insulin enables cells to absorb glucose from the bloodstream more efficiently. Insulin is a hormone that is essential for controlling blood sugar levels. Studies indicate that drinking green tea could improve insulin sensitivity, which could help people control their blood sugar levels.

THE PROPERTIES OF HIBISCUS TEA AS ANTIOXIDANTS

The bright petals of the hibiscus plant are used to make hibiscus tea, which is well known for its antioxidant qualities. Free radicals can cause oxidative stress and inflammation in the body, hence antioxidants are essential in countering their effects. The antioxidants in hibiscus tea have the potential to promote general health by reducing oxidative stress and perhaps affecting blood sugar management.

BLOOD SUGAR, RELAXATION, AND CHAMOMILE TEA

The relaxing properties of chamomile tea, which is made from the dried flowers of the chamomile plant, are frequently praised. Blood sugar levels can be affected by stress and sleep deprivation, and chamomile tea's relaxing qualities may help with blood sugar regulation inadvertently. Chamomile tea has the potential to be a beneficial supplement to a comprehensive strategy for sustaining stable blood sugar levels since it encourages relaxation and may lessen stress.

WARNINGS AND POINTS TO REMEMBER:

Even though drinking herbal teas may help control blood sugar, there are certain things to keep in mind when consuming them. Herbal teas can have different effects on different people. It is best to speak with a healthcare provider if you have any medical concerns or are on medication. Herbal teas should also be seen as a component of a holistic strategy that includes a healthy diet, frequent exercise, and other lifestyle choices rather than as the only remedy.

Adding herbal teas to one's routine, such as hibiscus, green, and chamomile teas, might be a tasty and possibly helpful approach to blood sugar control.

Comprehending the distinct characteristics of different teas, like the antioxidants in hibiscus tea or the catechins in green tea, sheds light on their potential health benefits. But it's important to drink herbal tea mindfully, taking into account personal health circumstances and, if necessary, consulting a professional.

CHAPTER SEVEN

INCLUDING HERBS IN YOUR NUTRITION

HERBAL EXTRACTS AND INFUSIONS

Including herbs in your diet can be a satisfying and all-encompassing way to keep your body healthy generally. Herbal infusions and extracts are among the most used ways to reap the health benefits of herbs. Herbs are steeped in hot water to release their medicinal compounds into the liquid, a process known as herbal infusion. This is a great way to enjoy the tastes and medicinal properties of different herbs, and it's similar to brewing a cup of tea.

CREATING INFUSIONS USING HERBS

Herbal infusion preparation is a simple procedure. To begin, cover the herbs with boiling water and steep for the recommended length of time. Depending on the herb and how it will be used, the duration may change. For example, infusions of chamomile are often drunk before bed to help with relaxation, while infusions of peppermint are well-known for helping with digestion.

MAKING HERBAL EXTRACTS

Herbal extracts provide a concentrated version of the plant's active ingredients in addition to infusions. To extract the medicinal qualities of the herbs, a solvent such as glycerin or alcohol is used. This concentrated liquid adds a strong dose of beneficial herbs to food or drinks. There are differences in extraction techniques, and for a more customized experience, some people choose to make their extracts at home.

SUPPLEMENTS WITH HERBS

Supplementing with herbs has become more and more popular as a convenient way to include herbs in daily life. These supplements, which are available in several formats like capsules, tablets, or tinctures, offer a convenient way to get the health benefits of herbs without having to prepare them in any way.

Nonetheless, to guarantee purity and potency, it's imperative to select premium supplements.

SELECTING HIGH-QUALITY SUPPLEMENTS

It's important to take into account various aspects while choosing herbal supplements, including the manufacturing method, the source of the herbs, and the use of fillers or additives. You may be sure that the decisions you make are in line with your health goals by choosing supplements from reliable brands or seeking advice from medical experts.

SPEAKING WITH MEDICAL EXPERTS

Speaking of medical professionals, you must speak with them before adding herbs to your diet, particularly if you use medication or have pre-existing medical conditions. Although most people consider herbs to be harmless, there is always a risk when they combine with specific drugs or diseases. Medical specialists can offer tailored guidance that considers your unique health profile and guides you through the possible advantages and disadvantages of using herbal supplements.

Finally, adding herbs to your diet through extracts, infusions, and supplements can be a tasty and nutritious experience. Through knowledge of how to prepare herbs, selecting premium supplements, and consulting medical professionals, you may take advantage of the many advantages that herbs can provide in terms of improving your general health.

CHAPTER EIGHT

BLOOD SUGAR CONTROL AND LIFESTYLE FACTORS

THE EFFECTS OF EXERCISE ON BLOOD SUGAR

Exercise is essential for controlling blood sugar levels and has several advantages for people with diabetes or those who are at risk of getting the disease. Regular exercise enhances insulin sensitivity, enabling cells to utilize glucose more effectively and react to insulin more effectively. Consequently, this helps to control blood sugar levels. It has been demonstrated that resistance training, such as weightlifting, and aerobic exercises, like walking, running, or swimming, are both beneficial in controlling blood sugar levels.

EXERCISE TYPES

Aerobic exercises improve cardiovascular health and aid in weight control, which is crucial for blood sugar regulation. These actions raise the body's need for glucose and encourage cells to absorb it so they can produce energy. Resistance training, on the other hand, promotes muscle growth, which enhances insulin sensitivity and glucose metabolism. It is frequently advised to incorporate both kinds of exercise into a well-rounded regimen for thorough blood sugar control.

HOW TO DESIGN A BALANCED WORKOUT PROGRAM

Developing a well-rounded workout plan requires taking into account several variables, such as the person's fitness level, preferences, and overall health. It's crucial to begin cautiously, particularly for newcomers or people with pre-existing medical conditions. Maintaining a regular schedule and including both resistance and aerobic training guarantees a comprehensive approach. Exercise regimens should be customized to an individual's capacity to maximize consistency and minimize the risk of injury or burnout.

STRESS REDUCTION

Another important lifestyle component that affects blood sugar regulation is stress management. Because stress hormones like cortisol cause the liver to produce glucose, prolonged stress can raise blood sugar levels. The application of efficacious stress management strategies is vital for persons who aspire to achieve blood sugar regulation. Methods like yoga, meditation, and deep breathing exercises can ease tension and foster serenity.

TECHNIQUES FOR RELAXATION AND MINDFULNESS

Techniques for relaxation and mindfulness are important components of the overall blood sugar control plan. For example, mindful eating encourages healthier eating practices by focusing on the tastes, textures, and feelings of food. Similar to this, relaxation methods like guided imagery or progressive muscle relaxation can lower tension and have a beneficial effect on blood sugar levels. Including these routines in daily life can help promote a more thoughtful and balanced attitude to health.

Effective blood sugar control requires a multimodal approach to lifestyle factors. Exercise is crucial since it has a variety of effects on insulin sensitivity and general health. The secret is to design a well-rounded fitness program that incorporates both resistance and aerobic training. Additionally, maintaining ideal blood sugar levels requires stress management using mindfulness and relaxation practices. People can actively participate in the management and prevention of problems associated with blood sugar regulation by adopting these components into their lifestyle.

CHAPTER NINE

KEEPING AN EYE ON AND SUSTAINING BLOOD SUGAR LEVELS

FREQUENT INSPECTION

Maintaining general health and effectively controlling diabetes need routine blood sugar testing. People with diabetes, especially those on insulin or oral drugs, should check their blood glucose levels frequently to assess the efficacy of their therapy and make any required modifications. A glucometer, a portable instrument that detects blood glucose levels from a small blood sample often acquired by pricking the fingertip, is used in this process.

GLUCOMETERS: THEIR APPLICATION

Glucometers are essential tools for people with diabetes daily. These gadgets offer a simple and quick way to check blood sugar levels while traveling or at home. A test strip is loaded with a tiny amount of blood, and the strip is put into the glucometer.

In a matter of seconds, the device analyzes the sample and shows the blood glucose level. When people and their healthcare providers use glucometers regularly, blood sugar changes can be monitored and decisions about medicine, nutrition, and lifestyle can be made with greater knowledge.

INTERPRETING THE OUTCOMES

Understanding the blood glucose monitoring data is essential for managing diabetes effectively. Stress, physical activity, and meals are some of the variables that can cause blood sugar levels to fluctuate throughout the day. Making educated decisions about their daily routines and spotting possible problems is made possible by comprehending the patterns and trends that glucose monitoring reveals. A medical expert can assist in interpreting the data and advising patients on how to modify their lifestyle or take their medications.

STRATEGIES FOR LONG-TERM MAINTENANCE

Maintaining appropriate blood sugar levels and avoiding diabetes-related problems require long-term management plans. A good long-term treatment plan consists of maintaining a healthy weight, taking medications as prescribed and engaging in regular physical activity. Regular check-ups with medical professionals also aid in keeping an eye on general health and addressing any new diabetes-related issues.

NUTRITIONAL ASPECTS

Blood sugar regulation is significantly influenced by dietary factors. For those who have diabetes, a well-balanced and managed diet is crucial. Crucial components of dietary control include keeping an eye on the amount of carbohydrates consumed, favoring complex carbs over simple sugars, and including a range of nutrient-dense meals. A certified dietician can offer individualized advice on developing a meal plan that supports stable blood sugar levels and is in line with personal health objectives.

SUSTAINING HERBAL ASSISTANCE

Apart from traditional methods, some people look into herbal help for managing their diabetes. Certain herbs may provide potential benefits, but it is best to approach herbs and supplements cautiously and in collaboration with a healthcare provider. Herbs like fenugreek and cinnamon, for instance, may lower blood sugar levels, according to certain research. However it's important to remember that herbal supplements may have negative effects or interfere with pharmaceuticals, so it's best to speak with a doctor before using them in a diabetic treatment plan.

Controlling blood sugar levels requires a multimodal approach that includes using glucometers regularly, interpreting the results, developing long-term maintenance plans, paying close attention to dietary restrictions, and, for some people, researching herbal support under a doctor's supervision. By improving general health and lowering the risk of consequences from uncontrolled blood sugar levels, these coordinated measures help to effectively manage diabetes.